Normal Pregnancy

Physiology and Management

Akmal El-Mazny

CONTENTS

INTRODUCTION

Pregnancy is a peculiar physiological state in which many changes take place to help adaptation of the woman's body to pregnancy.

Understanding these changes is essential for discrimination between normal pregnancy symptoms and pathological conditions, and for understanding the effect of pregnancy on preexisting diseases.

Although pregnancy is considered a normal physiological event, yet it may be complicated by a disease or a disorder that affects the health or endangers the life of the mother or the fetus.

Antenatal care is a program of preventive obstetrics, with a main objective to ensure a safe motherhood, culminating in a safe delivery of a healthy fetus.

This book provides a comprehensive review of normal pregnancy, emphasizing its physiology and management, which will be of immense value for obstetricians and allied health professionals.

By developing a clear understanding of what is normal, you will better understand abnormalities affecting pregnancy and the rationale behind treatment.

GAMETES

Pregnancy occurs when a mature liberated ovum is fertilized by a mature capacitated spermatozoon.

GAMETOGENESIS

Primitive germ cells are present in the embryo by the end of the third week.

They start to migrate via the dorsal mesentery and reach the indifferent gonad by the end of the fourth week of development.

Gametogenesis reduces the number of chromosomes to half and alters the shape of germ cells to suit their functions.

Steps of Gametogenesis

Proliferation: of germ cells into daughter gonocytes by mitosis.

Growth: of some daughter gonocytes into primary gonocytes.

Maturation: First maturation division is a reduction division with long prophase and second maturation division with no prophase.

Oogenesis starts in utero and is arrested in the prophase for years to be completed just before ovulation, while spermatogenesis starts at puberty and continues indefinitely.

In oogenesis only one mature ovum is produced from an oocyte.

THE OVUM

The ovum leaves the ovary after rupture of the Graafian follicle, carrying 23 chromosomes and surrounded by the zona pellucida and corona radiata.

The ovum is picked up by the fimbriated end of the Fallopian tubes and moved towards the ampulla by the ciliary movement of the cells and rhythmic peristalsis of the tube.

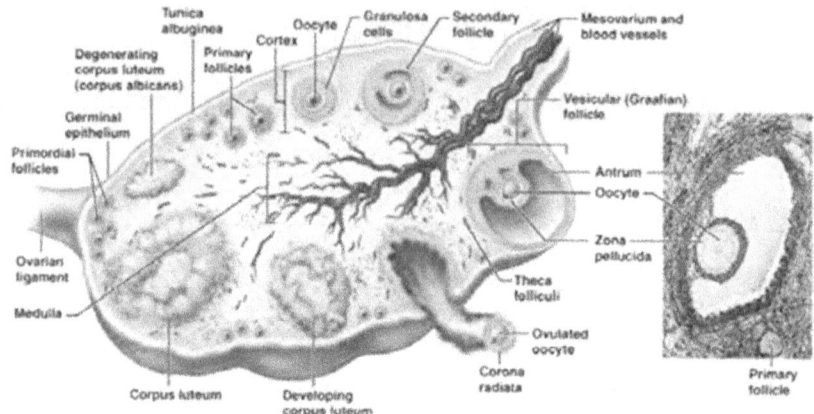

Mature Ovum

THE SPERM

The spermatozoa leave the testis carrying 23 chromosomes but not yet capable of fertilization.

Their maturation is completed through their journey in the epididymis and when mixed with the seminal plasma from the epididymis, seminal vesicle and prostate gland.

After semen is ejaculated, the sperms reach the cervix by their own motility within seconds leaving behind the seminal plasma in the vagina.

At time of ovulation, the cervical mucous is in the most favourable condition for sperm penetration and capacitation as:

- It becomes more copious, less viscous and its macromolecules arrange in parallel chains providing channels for sperms passage.

- Its contents from glucose and chloride are increased.

The sperms ascent through the uterine cavity and Fallopian tubes to reach the site of fertilization in the ampulla by:

- Its own motility.

- Uterine and tubal peristalsis (aggravated by seminal prostaglandins).

The sperms reach the tube within 30-40 minutes but they are capable of fertilization after 2-6 hours; this period is needed for sperm capacitation.

Capacitation of sperms is the process after which the sperm becomes able to penetrate the zona pellucida, that surrounding the ovum and fertilize it.

The cervical and tubal secretions are mainly responsible for this capacitation.

Capacitation is believed to be due to:

– Increase in the DNA concentration in the nucleus.

– Increase permeability of the coat of sperm head to allow more release of hyaluronidase.

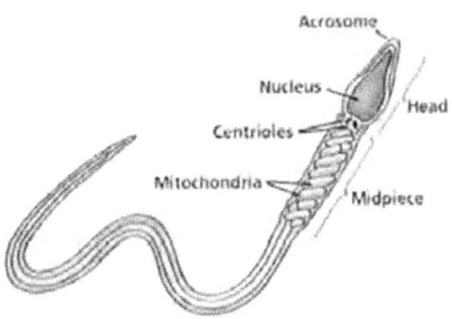

Mature Sperm

FERTILIZATION

Fertilization is the fusion of male and female pronuclei.

Millions of sperms ejaculated in the vagina, but only hundreds of thousands reach the outer portion of the tubes.

Only few succeed to penetrate the zona pellucida, and only one spermatozoon enters the ovum transversing the perivitelline space.

STEPS OF FERTILIZATION

Zona Binding: The sperm head binds to zona pellucida associated with acrosomal reaction and release of acrosomal enzymes.

Zona Penetration: This is facilitated by acrosomal release.

Oolemmal Fusion: Oolemmal fusion is facilitated by integrin B1-6.

After penetration of the ovum by a sperm, the zona pellucida resists penetration by another sperms due to alteration of its electrical potential.

The pronucleus of both ovum and sperm unite together to form the zygote (46 chromosomes).

SEX DETERMINATION

The ovum carries 22 autosomes and one X chromosome, while the sperm carries 22 autosomes and either an X or Y chromosome.

If the sperm is carrying X chromosome the baby will be a female (46 XX), if it is carrying Y chromosome the baby will be a male (46 XY).

CLEAVAGE AND BLASTOCYST FORMATION

On its way to the uterine cavity, the fertilized ovum (zygote) divides into 2, 4, 8 then 16 cells (blastomeres).

This division (cleavage) starts within 24 hours of fertilization and occurs nearly every 12 hours repeatedly.

The resultant 16 cells mass is called "morula" which reaches the uterine cavity after about 4 days from fertilization.

A cavity appears within the morula converting it into a cystic structure called "blastocyst" in which the cells become arranged into:

– An inner mass (embryoblast) which will form the embryo.

– An outer layer (trophoblast) which invade the uterine wall.

The blastocyst remains free in the uterine cavity for 3-4 days, during which it is nourished by the secretion of the endometrium (uterine milk).

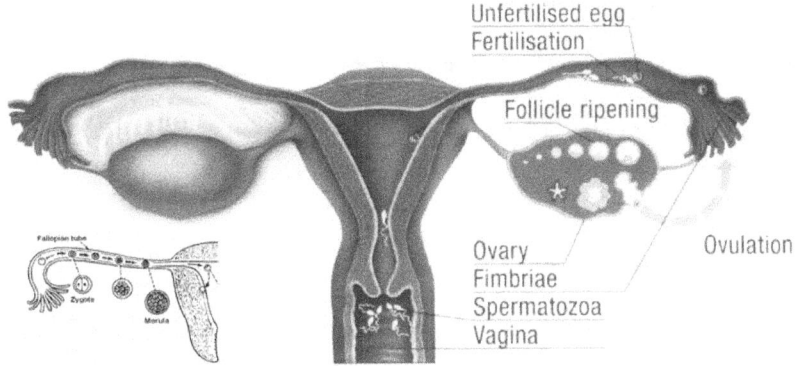

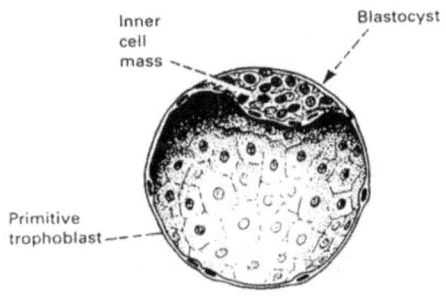

Cleavage and Blastocyst Formation

IMPLANTATION

Implantation is imbedding of fertilized ovum in the uterine mucosa.

DECIDUA

It is the thickened vascular endometrium of the pregnant uterus.

It is called so because it casts of after parturition.

The glands become enlarged, tortuous and filled with secretion.

The stroma cells become large with small nuclei and clear cytoplasm, these are called decidual cells.

The decidua, like secretory endometrium, consists of three layers:

– Superficial compact layer.

– Intermediate spongy layer.

– Thin basal layer.

The separation of placenta occurs through the spongy layer while the endometrium regenerates again from the basal layer.

The trophoblast of the blastocyst invades the decidua to be implanted in:

– The posterior surface of the upper uterine segment in about 2/3 of cases.

– The anterior surface of the upper uterine segment in about 1/3 of cases.

STAGES OF IMPLANTATION

Apposition of Blastocyst: This is a close contact brought about by pinocytosis of uterine fluid, and the glandular crypts of secretory endometrium.

Adhesion of Trophoblast: The zona pellucida disappears and the blastocyst hatches, out to come in contact with the surface uterine epithelium.

Invasion of the Trophoblast: Trophoblastic invasion is brought about by a variety of proteases secreted by trophoblast.

After implantation the decidua becomes differentiated into:

– Decidua basalis: under the site of implantation.

– Decidua capsularis: covering the ovum.

– Decidua parietalis or vera: lining the rest of the uterine cavity.

As the conceptus enlarges and fills the uterine cavity the decidua capsularis fuses with the decidua parietalis nearly at the end of 12 weeks.

The decidua has the following functions:

– It is the site of implantation.

– It resists more invasion of the trophoblast.

– It nourishes the early implanted ovum by its glycogen and lipid contents.

– It shares in the formation of the placenta.

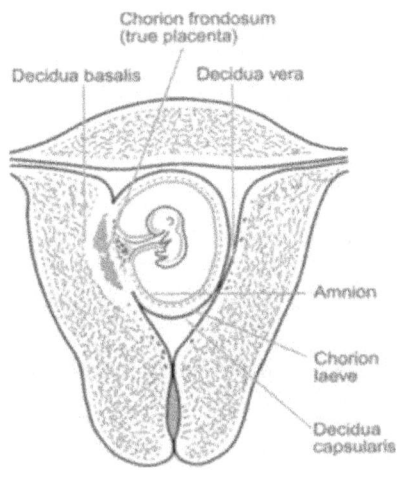

Decidua

DEVELOPMENT OF BLASTOCYST

Outer Trophoblast Layer (Chorion)

After implantation, the trophoblast differentiates into 2 layers:

– An outer one called syncytium (syncytiotrophoblast) which is multinucleated cells without cell boundaries,

– An inner one called Langhan's layer (cytotrophoblast) which is cuboidal cells with simple cytoplasm.

A third layer of mesoderm appears inner to the cytotrophoblast.

The trophoblast and the lining mesoderm together form the chorion.

Mesodermal tissue (connecting stalk) connects the inner cell mass to the chorion and will form the umbilical cord later on.

Spaces (lacunae) appear in the syncytium, increase in size and fuse together to form the "chorio-decidual space" or "intervillus space".

Erosion of the decidual blood vessels by the trophoblast allows blood to circulate in this space.

The outer syncytium and inner Langhan's cells form buds surrounding the developing ovum called "primary villi".

When the mesoderm invades the center of the primary villi they are called "secondary villi".

When blood vessels (branches from the umbilical vessels) develop inside the mesodermal core, they are called "tertiary villi".

At first, the chorionic villi surround the developing ovum.

After the 12th week, the villi opposite the decidua capsularis atrophy leaving the chorion laeve which forms the outer layer of the fetal membrane and is attached to the margin of the placenta.

The villi opposite the decidua basalis grow and branch to form the chorion frondosum and together with the decidua basalis will form the placenta.

Some of these villi attach to the decidua basalis (the basal plate) called the "anchoring villi".

Other villi hang freely in the intervillous spaces called the "absorbing villi"

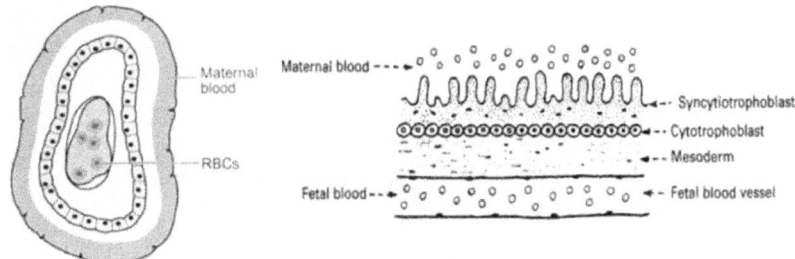

Tertiary Villi

Inner Cell Mass

After implantation, 2 cavities appear in the inner cell mass:

– The amniotic cavity.

– The yolk sac.

In-between these 2 cavities the mesoderm develops.

The layer of cells at the floor of the amniotic cavity will give the ectodermal structures of the fetus.

The layer of cells at the roof of the yolk sac will give the endodermal structures of the fetus.

The mesoderm inbetween will give the mesodermal structure.

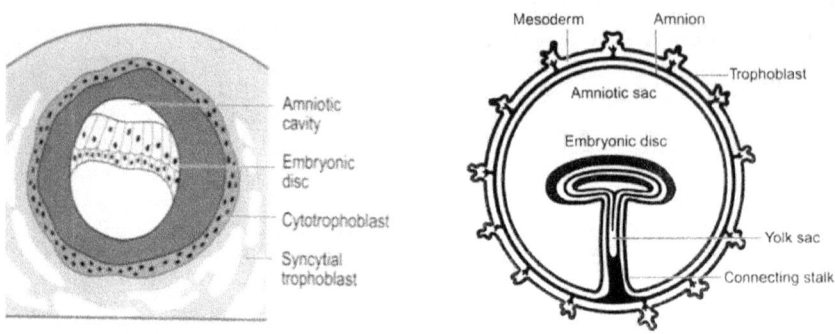

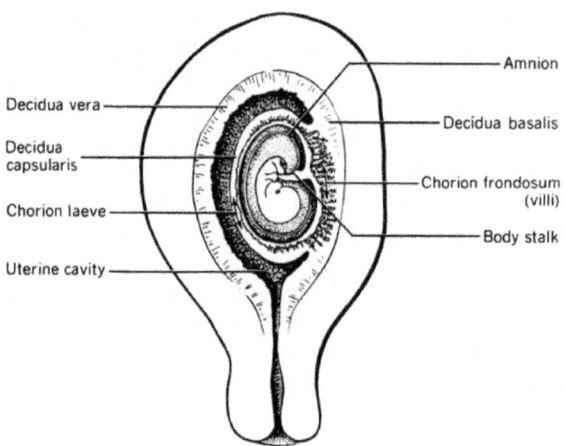

Inner Cell Mass

EMBRYO DEVELOPMENT

Some of the major hallmarks of embryologic development are noted here in developmental weeks.

To correlate with gestational age, adjust by adding 2 weeks to account for time from the last menstrual period to fertilization.

WEEKS (3-8)

The period of organogenesis.

It is critical for normal development.

It is the time when most structural birth defects occur.

WEEK (4)

The neural tube closes.

WEEK (5)

– Limb and facial development begin.

– The embryo appears tightly C-shaped.

WEEK (6)

– Early formation of fingers and toes.

– Brain vesicles are prominent.

– The external ear forms.

– Umbilical herniation begins, caused by swelling from intestinal loops in the umbilical cord and is a normal embryologic event.

– Midgut herniation at this gestational age should not be confused with an omphalocele, which is the abnormal herniation of abdominal organs through an enlarged umbilical ring.

WEEK (7)

– Pigmentation of the retina is seen.

– Fingers and toes separate.

– The upper lip and nipples form.

WEEK (8)

– Limbs are long and bent at the elbows and knees.

– The face is more human-like.

– The tail disappears.

WEEKS (11-13)

– The bowel returns to the abdominal cavity.

– The long bones and skull ossify.

– The embryo is called a fetus at the 8th gestational week.

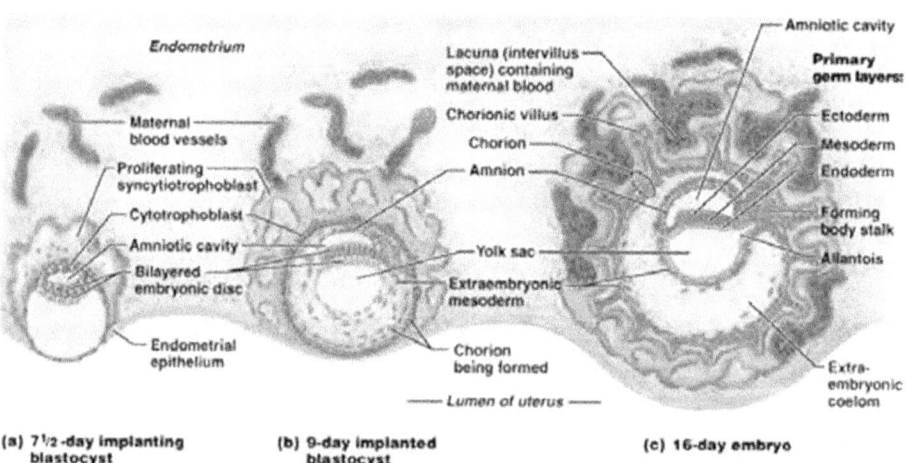

Early Embryo Development

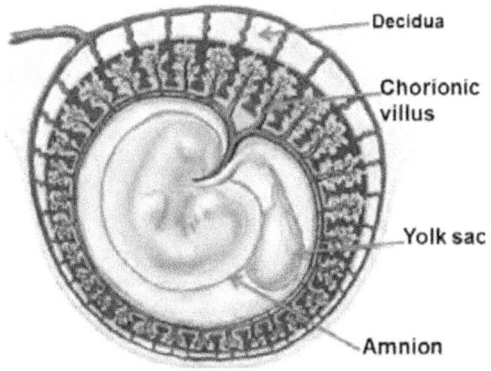

Decidua

Chorionic villus

Yolk sac

Amnion

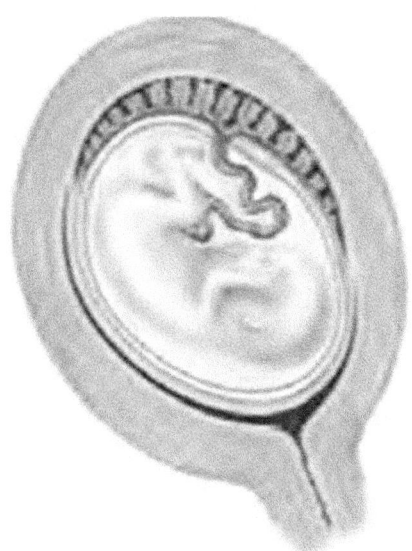

Late Fetal Development

PLACENTA

ANATOMY

Origin

The placenta develops from:

– Chorion frondosum (fetal origin).

– Decidua basalis (maternal origin).

Shape: discoid.

Diameter: 15-20 cm.

Weight: 500 gm.

Thickness: 2.5 cm at its center and gradually tapers towards the periphery.

Position: in the upper uterine segment (99.5%), either in the posterior surface (2/3) or the anterior surface (1/3).

Surfaces

Fetal Surface

Smooth, glistening and is covered by the amnion which is reflected on the cord.

The umbilical cord is inserted near or at the center of this surface and its radiating branches can be seen beneath the amnion.

Maternal Surface

Dull greyish red in colour and is divided into 15-20 cotyledons.

Each cotyledon is formed of the branches of one main villus stem covered by decidua basalis.

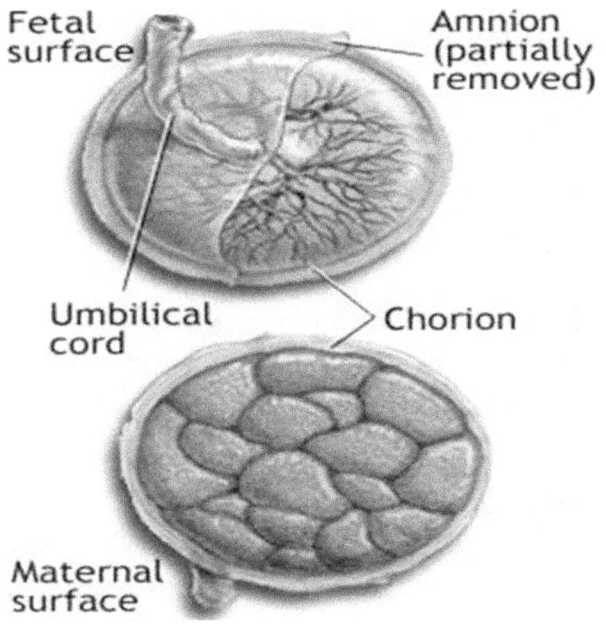

Placental Surfaces

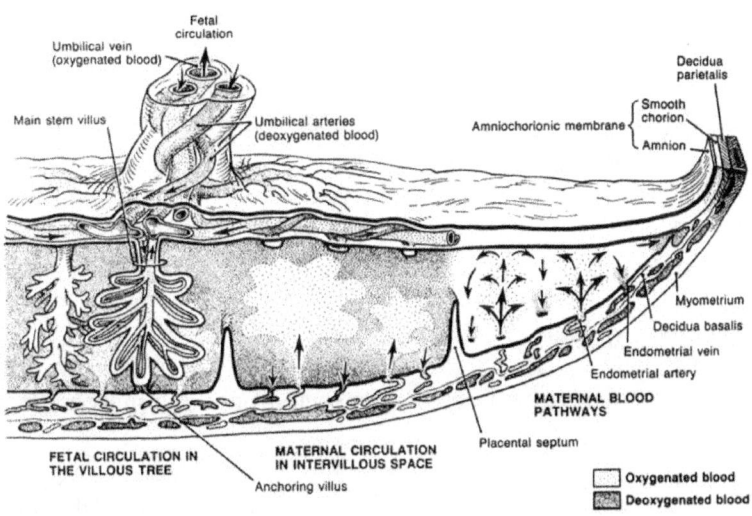

Placental Circulation

ABNORMALITIES OF THE PLACENTA

Abnormal Shape

Placenta Bilobata

The placenta consists of two equal lobes connected by placental tissue.

Placenta Bipartita

The placenta consists of two equal parts connected by membranes.

The umbilical cord is inserted in one lobe and branches from its vessels cross the membranes to the other lobe.

Rarely, the umbilical cord divides into two branches, each supplies a lobe.

Placenta Succenturiata

The placenta consists of a large lobe and a smaller one connecting together by membranes.

The umbilical cord is inserted into the large lobe and branches of its vessels cross the membranes to the small succenturiate (accessory) lobe.

The accessory lobe may be retained in the uterus after delivery leading to postpartum hemorrhage.

This is suspected if a circular gap is detected in the membranes from which blood vessels pass towards the edge of the main placenta.

Placenta Circumvallata

A whitish ring composed of decidua, is seen around the placenta from its fetal surface.

This may result when the chorion frondosum is two small for the nutrition of the fetus, so the peripheral villi grow in such a way splitting the decidua basalis into a superficial layer (the whitish ring) and a deep layer.

It can be a cause of abortion, antepartum hemorrhage, premature labor and intrauterine fetal death.

Placenta Fenestrata

A gap is seen in the placenta covered by membranes giving the appearance of a window.

Placenta Membranacea

A great part of the chorion develops into placental tissue.

The placenta is large, thin and may measure 30-40 cm in diameter.

It may encroach on the lower uterine segment i.e. placenta previa.

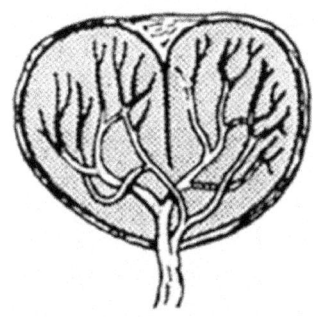   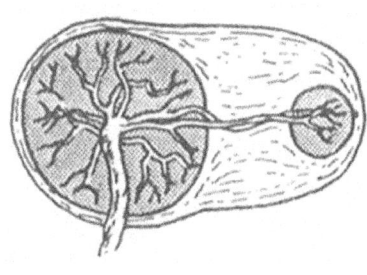

Placenta Bilobata   **Placenta Succenturiata**

Abnormal Weight

The placenta increases in size and weight as in:

– Congenital syphilis.

– Hydrops fetalis.

– Diabetes mellitus.

Abnormal Position

Placenta Previa

The placenta is partly or completely attached to lower uterine segment.

Abnormal Adhesion

Placenta Accreta

The chorionic villi penetrate deeply into the uterine wall to reach the myometrium, due to deficient decidua basalis.

When the villi penetrate deeply into the myometrium, it is called "placenta increta".

When they reach the peritoneal coat it is called "placenta percreta".

Placental Infarcts

White Infracts

Due to excessive fibrin deposition.

Normal placenta may contain white infracts in which calcium deposition may occur.

Red Infarcts

Due to hemorrhage from the maternal vessels of the decidua mainly in hypertensive states with pregnancy.

Old red infarcts finally become white due to fibrin deposition.

Placental Tumor

Chorioangioma

A rare benign tumor of the placental blood vessels.

May be associated with hydramnios.

FUNCTIONS OF THE PLACENTA

Barrier Function

The fetal blood in the chorionic villi is separated from the maternal blood, in the intervillous spaces, by the placental barrier which is composed of:

– Endothelium of the fetal blood vessels.

– Villous stroma.

– Cytotrophoblast.

– Syncytiotrophoblast.

However, it is an incomplete barrier; it allows the passage of antibodies (Ig G only), hormones, antibiotics, sedatives, some viruses as rubella and smallpox and some organisms as treponema pallida.

Substances of large molecular size as heparin and insulin cannot pass the placental barrier.

Respiratory Function

O2 and CO2 pass across the placenta by simple diffusion.

The fetal hemoglobin has more affinity and carrying capacity than adult hemoglobin.

2,3 diphosphoglycerate (2,3-DPG) which competes for oxygen binding sites in the hemoglobin molecule, is less bounded to the fetal hemoglobin (Hb F) and thereby allows a greater uptake of O2 (O2 affinity).

The rate of diffusion depends upon:

– Maternal/fetal gases gradient.

– Maternal and fetal placental blood flow.

– Placental permeability.

– Placental surface area.

Nutritive Function

The transfer of nutrients from the mother to the fetus is achieved by:

– Simple diffusion: e.g. water and electrolytes.

– Facilitated diffusion: e.g. glucose.

– Active diffusion: e.g. aminoacids.

– Pinocytosis: e.g. large protein molecules and cells.

Excretory Function

Waste products of the fetus as urea are passed to maternal blood by simple diffusion through the placenta.

Production of Enzymes

e.g. oxytocinase, monoamino oxidase, insulinase, histaminase and heat stable alkaline phosphatase.

Production of Proteins

Pregnancy associated plasma proteins (PAPP), e.g. PAPP-A, PAPP-B, PAPP-C, PAPP-D and PP5.

The exact function of these proteins is not defined.

Endocrine Function

Human Chorionic Gonadotrophin (hCG)

It is a glycoprotein produced by the syncytiotrophoblast.

It supports the corpus luteum in the first 10 weeks of pregnancy until the syncytiotrophoblast can produce progesterone.

hCG molecule is composed of 2 subunits:

– Alpha subunit which is similar to that of FSH, LH and TSH.

– Beta subunit which is specific to hCG.

hCG rises sharply after implantation, reaches a peak of 100000 mIU/ml about the 60th day of pregnancy then falls sharply by the day 100 to 30000 mIU/ml and is maintained at this level until term.

Estimation of B-hCG is used for:

– Diagnosis of early pregnancy.

– Diagnosis of ectopic pregnancy.

– Diagnosis and flow-up of trophoblastic disease.

Estrogens

They are synthetized by syncytiotrophoblast from their precursors dehydroepiandrosterone sulphate (DHES) or its 16α-hydroxy (16α-OH-DHES).

Near term, 50% of DHES is drived from the fetal adrenal gland and 50% from maternal adrenal.

It is transformed in the placenta into estradiol- 17β (E2).

On the other hand, 90% of 16α-OH-DHES is drived from fetal origin after hydroxylation of DHES in the fetal liver, while only 10% is drived from the mother by the same way.

Estrogens are excreted in the maternal urine as estriol (E3), estradiol (E2) and estrone (E1). Estriol (E3) is the largest portion of them.

Maternal urinary and serum estriol level is an important index for fetal wellbeing as its synthesis depends mainly on the integrity of the fetal adrenal and liver as well as the placenta (feto-placental unit).

Urinary estriol increases as pregnancy advances to reach 35-40 mg per 24 hours at full term.

Progressive fall in urinary estriol indicates that the fetus is jeopardous.

Estrogens are responsible with progesterone for the most of the maternal changes due to pregnancy especially that in genital tract and breasts.

Progesterone

It is synthetized by syncytiotrophoblast from the maternal cholesterol.

Excreted in maternal urine as pregnandiol.

Increasing gradually during pregnancy to reach a daily production of 250 mg per day in late normal single pregnancy.

It provides a precursor for the fetal adrenal to produce glucocorticoids and mineralocorticoids.

Human Placental Lactogen (hPL)

It is a polypeptide hormone produced by the syncytiotrophoblast.

The supposed actions of hPL include:

– Lipolysis: increasing free fatty acids which provide a source of energy for mother and fetal nutrition.

– Inhibition of gluconeogenesis: thus spare both glucose and protein explaining the anti-insulin effect of hPL.

– Somatotrophic: i.e. growth promotion of the fetus due to increased supply of fatty acids, glucose and amino acids.

– Mammotropic and lactogenic effect.

HPL can be detected by the 5-6th week of pregnancy, rises steadily until the 36th week to be 6m g/ml.

Its level is proportional to the placental mass.

Human Chorionic Thyrotrophin (hCT)

No significant role has been established for it.

It is probably responsible for increased maternal thyroid activity and promotion of fetal thyroid development.

Hypothalamic and Pituitary Like Hormones

e.g. gonadotropin releasing hormone (GnRH), corticotropin releasing factor (CRF), ACTH and melanocyte stimulating hormone (MSH).

Others

e.g. inhibin, relaxin and beta endorphins.

Immunological Function

The placenta appears to be an important factor in maternal acceptance of the fetus.

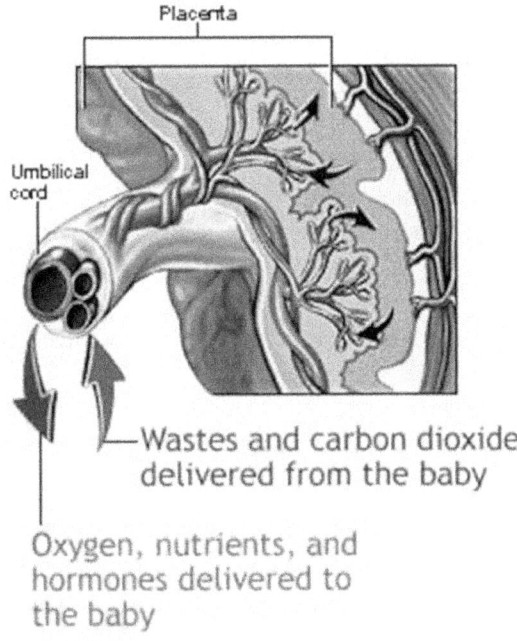

Placental Functions

UMBILICAL CORD

ANATOMY

Origin: It develops from the connecting stalk.

Length: At term, it measures about 50 cm.

Diameter: 2 cm.

Insertion: in the fetal surface of the placenta near the center "eccentric insertion" (70%) or at the center "central insertion" (30%).

Structure

It consists of mesodermal connective tissue called Wharton's jelly, covered by amnion.

It contains:

- One umbilical vein carries oxygenated blood from the placenta to the fetus.

- Two umbilical arteries carry deoxygenated blood from the fetus to the placenta.

- Remnants of the yolk sac and allantois.

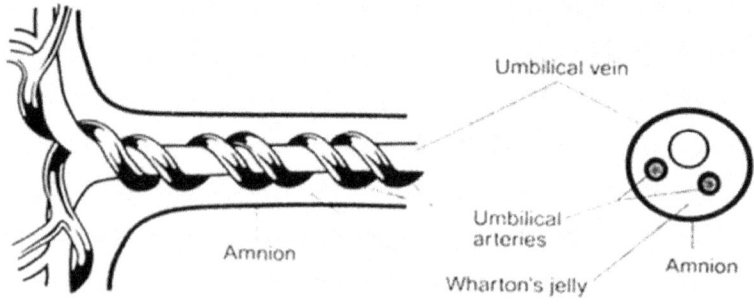

Structure of the Umbilical Cord

ABNORMALITIES OF THE UMBILICAL CORD

Abnormal Cord Insertion

<u>Marginal Insertion:</u> in the placenta (battledore insertion).

<u>Velamentous Insertion:</u> in the membranes and vessels connect the cord to the edge of the placenta.

If these vessels pass at the region of the internal os, the condition is called "vasa previa".

Vasa previa can occur also when the vessels connecting a succenturiate lobe with the main placenta pass at the region of the internal os.

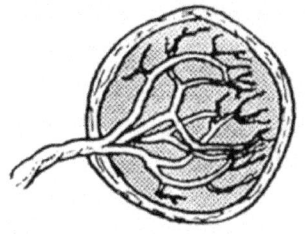 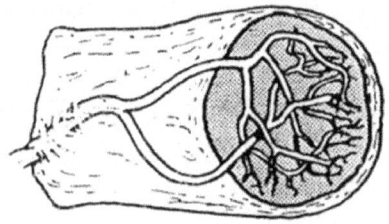

Marginal Insertion   **Velamentous Insertion**

Abnormal Cord Length

<u>Long Cord</u>

This may lead to:

– Cord presentation.

– Cord prolapse.

– Coiling of the cord around the neck.

– True knots of the cord.

Short Cord

May be:

– True.

– Apparent (due to coiling of the cord around the neck).

This may lead to:

– Intrapartum hemorrhage due to premature separation of the placenta.

– Delayed descent of the fetus during labor.

– Inversion of the uterus.

Knots of the Cord

True Knot

When the fetus passes through a loop of the cord.

If pulled tight, fetal asphyxia may result.

False Knot

Localised collection of Wharton's jelly.

Containing a loop of umbilical vessels.

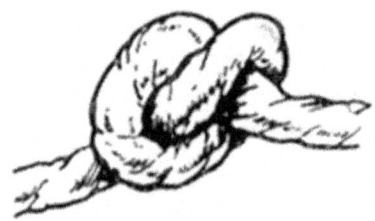
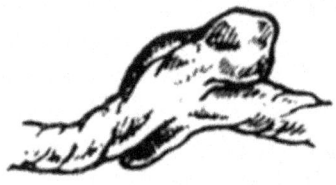

True Knot   **False Knot**

Torsion of the Cord

It may occur particularly in the portion near the fetus where the Wharton's jelly is less abundant.

Hematoma

Due to rupture of one of the umbilical vessels.

Single Umbilical Artery

It may be associated with other fetal congenital anomalies.

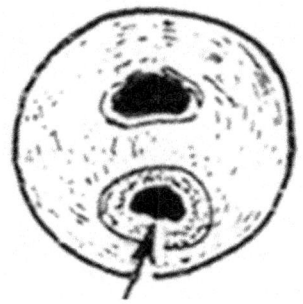

Single Umbilical Artery

FETAL MEMBRANES

THE CHORION

Is the outer membrane.

It is in contact with the uterine wall.

It is attached to the margins of the placenta.

Histologically, it is composed of 4 layers:

– Cellular layer.

– Dense reticulum.

– Pseudo-basement membrane.

– Outer trophoblast.

THE AMNION

Is a transparent greyish membrane which lines the chorion.

It covers the fetal surface of the placenta and the umbilical cord.

The amniotic sac contains the fetus swimming in the liquor amnii.

Histologically, it is composed of 5 layers:

– Cellular layer.

– Basement membrane.

– Compact layer.

– Fibroblast layer.

– Outer spongy layer adherent to the cellular layer of the chorion.

AMNIOTIC FLUID

NATURE

It is a clear pale, slightly alkaline (pH 7.2) fluid.

It is about 400 ml at mid pregnancy, reaches about 1000 ml at 36-38 weeks then decreases later on to be scanty in post-term pregnancy.

ORIGIN

Fetal

– Active secretion from the amniotic epithelium.

– Transudation from the fetal circulation.

– Fetal urine.

Maternal

Transudation from maternal circulation.

CIRCULATION

Uptake of amniotic fluid is by absorption through the amnion to the maternal circulation and by fetal swallowing.

COMPOSITION

– Water (98-99%).

– Carbohydrates (glucose and fructose), proteins (albumin and globulins), lipids, hormones (estrogen and progesterone), enzymes (alkaline phosphatase).

– Minerals (sodium, potassium and chloride).

– Suspended materials as vernix caseosa, lanugo hair, desquamated epithelial cells and meconium.

FUNCTIONS

During Pregnancy

– Protects the fetus against injury.

– A medium for free fetal movement.

– Maintains the fetal temperature.

– Source for nutrition of the fetus.

– A medium for fetal excretion.

During Labor

– The fore-bag of water helps the dilatation of the cervix during labor.

– It acts as an antiseptic for the birth canal after rupture of the membranes.

FETAL CIRCULATION

BEFORE BIRTH

The umbilical vein carries oxygenated blood from the placenta to the fetus.

It divides into a branch joining the portal vein and another joining the inferior vena cava to the right atrium (ductus venosus).

Most blood of the right atrium passes through the foramen ovale to the left atrium, left ventricle to the aorta.

Some blood of the right atrium passes to the right ventricle to the pulmonary artery, but most of this blood is directed to the aorta through the ductus arteriosus.

The 2 umbilical arteries (branches of internal iliac "hypogastric artery") carry deoxygenated blood from the fetus to the placenta.

AFTER BIRTH

The following changes occur:

– Due to ligation of the umbilical cord, the large volume of blood returning to the fetus through the umbilical vein stops, hence venous pressure falls in the inferior vena cava causing the ductus venosus to close and becomes the ligamentum venosum later on.

– Neonatal respiration creates a negative intrathoracic pressure which opens the pulmonary capillary bed leading to falling of the pressure in the right atrium while that in the left atrium is increased due to increased amount of blood returning from the pulmonary veins, thus causing functional closure of the foramen ovale (closes anatomically after 1 year).

– With diversion of most of the blood into the lungs and increased oxygen concentration, the ductus arteriosus contracts (prostaglandin mediated) and becomes obliterated to form the ligamentum arteriosum later on.

– The umbilical vein is obliterated to form the ligamentum teres and the distal ends of the fetal hypogastric arteries are obliterated to form the hypogastric ligaments (lateral umbilical ligaments).

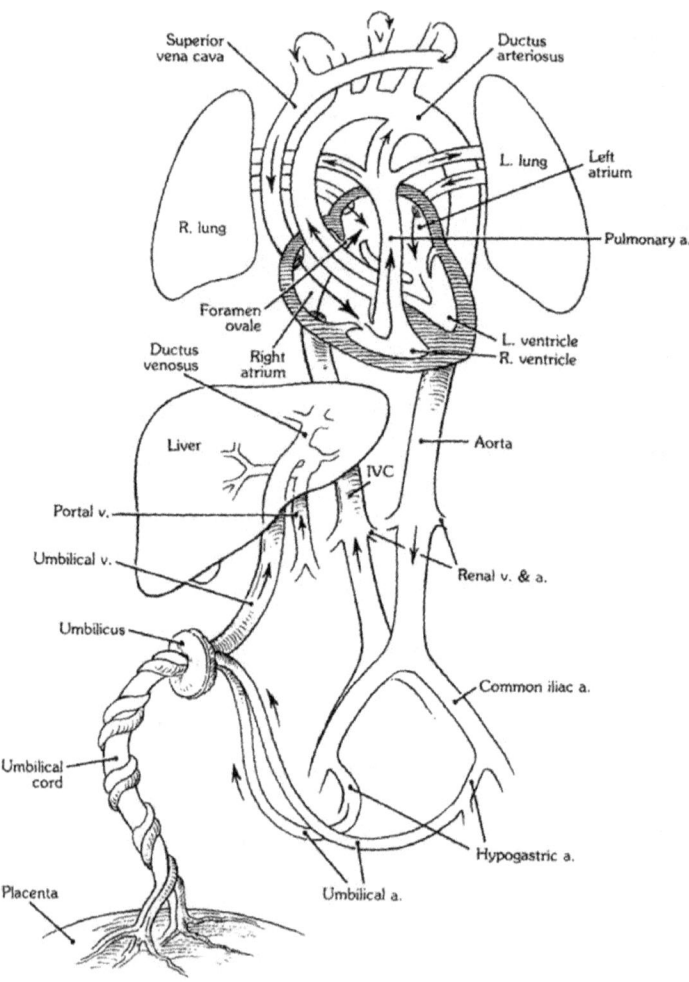

Fetal Circulation

MATERNAL CHANGES DURING PREGNANCY

GENITAL CHANGES

The Uterus

Size: increases from 7.5 x 5 x 2.5 cm in non-pregnant state to 35 x 25 x 20 cm at term.

Weight: increases from 50 gm in non-pregnant state to 1000 gm at term. This is due to:

- Hypertrophy of the muscle fibres (estrogen effect) and their multiplication (progesterone effect).

- Increase in the mass of elastic connective tissue.

Capacity: increases from 4 ml in non-pregnant state to 4000 ml at term.

Shape: becomes globular by the 8th week and pyriform by the 16th week till term.

Position: with ascent from the pelvis, the uterus usually undergoes rotation with tilting to the right (dextro-rotation), probably due to presence of the rectosigmoid colon on the left side.

Consistency: becomes progressively softer due to:

- Increased vascularity.

- Presence of amniotic fluid.

Contractility

From the first trimester onwards, the uterus undergoes irregular contractions called Braxton Hicks Contractions, which normally are painless.

They may cause some discomfort late in pregnancy and may account for false labor pain.

Utero-Placental Blood Flow

Uterine and ovarian vessels increase in diameter, length and tortuosity.

Uterine blood flow increases progressively and reaches about 500 ml/minute at term.

Formation of Lower Uterine Segment

After 12 weeks, the isthmus (0.5cm) starts to expand gradually to form the lower uterine segment which measures 10 cm in length at term.

	Upper Uterine Segment	Lower Uterine Segment
Peritoneum	Firmly-attached.	Loosely-attached.
Myometrium	3 layers: - Outer longitudinal. - Middle oblique. - Inner circular.	2 layers: - Outer longitudinal. - Inner circular.
Activity	Active: Contracts, retracts and becomes thicker during labor.	Passive: Dilates, stretches and becomes thinner during labor.
Decidua	Well-developed.	Poorly-developed.
Membranes	Firmly-attached.	Loosely-attached.

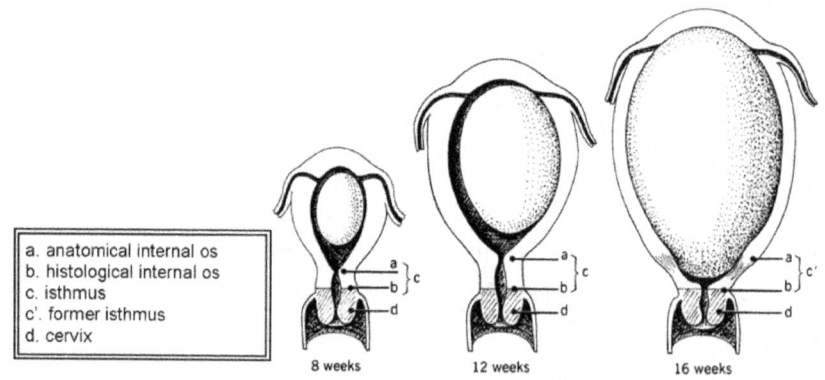

a. anatomical internal os
b. histological internal os
c. isthmus
c'. former isthmus
d. cervix

8 weeks   12 weeks   16 weeks

Lower Uterine Segment

The Cervix

It becomes hypertrophied, soft and bluish in colour due to edema and increased vascularity.

Soon after conception, a thick cervical secretion obstructs the cervical canal forming a mucous plug.

The endocervical epithelium proliferates and/or everted forming cervical ectopy (previously called erosion).

The Vagina

The vagina becomes soft, warm, moist with increased secretion and violet in colour (Chadwick's sign) due to increased vascularity.

The Vulva

It becomes soft, violet in colour.

Edema and varicosities may develop.

The Ovaries

Both ovaries are enlarged due to increased vascularity and edema particularly that containing the corpus luteum.

Corpus luteum starts to degenerate after the 10th week when the placenta is formed.

Corpus luteum secretes estrogen, progesterone and relaxin.

Relaxin is a protein hormone. Its exact role in pregnancy is unknown. It may induce softness and effacement of the cervix.

Ovulation ceases during pregnancy due to pituitary inhibition by the high levels of estrogen and progesterone.

The Fallopian Tubes

The musculature hypertrophies, and the epithelium becomes flattened.

BREAST CHANGES

In the early weeks, the pregnant woman experiences tenderness and tingling of the breasts.

After the second month the breasts increase in size and become nodular as a result of hypertrophy of the mammary alveoli.

Delicate veins become visible beneath the skin.

Pigmentation

The nipples become larger, deeply pigmented and more erectile.

The primary areola becomes deeply pigmented.

During the fifth month, a pigmented area appears around the primary areola called secondary areola.

Montgomery's Follicles

Hypertrophic sebaceous glands appear as non-pigmented elevations in the primary areola.

Colostrum

Thick yellowish fluid can be expressed from the nipples.

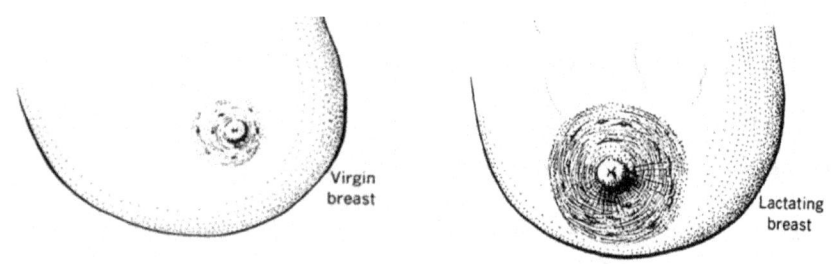

Breast Changes

SKIN CHANGES

Pigmentation

This is due to increased production of melanocyte stimulating hormone (MSH).

Chloasma Gravidarum (Pregnancy Mask)

A butterfly pigmentation appears on the checks and nose.

It usually disappears few months after labor.

Breasts

Increased pigmentation of the nipples and primary areolae and appearance of the secondary areolae.

Linea Nigra

A dark line extending from the umbilicus to the symphysis pubis.

Striae Gravidarum

These are reddish, slightly depressed streaks appear in the later months of pregnancy in the abdomen and sometimes breasts and thighs.

It may be due to mechanical stretching or increased glucocorticoids which results in rupture of the elastic fibres in the dermis and exposure of the vascular subcutaneous tissues.

After delivery, they become white in colour but do not disappear and called "striae albicans".

Vascular Changes

There is increase in the skin blood flow and temperature.

Secretions

Increase in sweat and sebaceous glands activity.

Loss of Hair

Sometimes occurs.

HEMATOLOGIC CHANGES

Blood Volume

The total blood volume increases steadily from early pregnancy to reach a maximum of 35-45% above the non-pregnant level at 32 weeks.

Plasma volume increases by 40% whereas red cell mass increases by 20% leading to hemodilution (Physiological anemia).

Blood Indices

Erythrocytes

Decrease during pregnancy from 4.5 millions to 3.7 millions /mm3 relative to the increase in plasma volume.

Its contents from 2, 3 diphosphoglycerate increase which competes for oxygen binding sites in the hemoglobin molecule thus release more O2 to the fetus.

Hemoglobin Concentration

Falls from 14 gm/dl to 12 gm/dl.

Erythrocyte Sedimentation Rate

Increases from 12 to 50 mm/hour.

Leucocytes

Increases from 7000/mm3 to 10.500/mm during pregnancy and up to 16000/mm3 during labor.

Fibrinogen

Increases from 200-400 mg/dl to 400-600 mg/dl.

CARDIOVASCULAR CHANGES

Heart

Position

As the diaphragm is elevated progressively during pregnancy the apex is displaced upwards and to the left so that it lies in the 4th intercostal space outside the midclavicular line.

Rate

The resting pulse rate increases by 10-15 beats per minute during pregnancy.

Cardiac Output

Increases mainly by increased stroke volume rather than increased heart rate reaching a maximum of 40% above the non-pregnant level at 20 weeks to be maintained till term.

During labor cardiac output increases more, particularly during the second stage due to pain, uterine contractions and expulsive efforts pushing the blood into the general circulation.

Postpartum, the increased cardiac output is maintained for up to 4 days and then declines rapidly.

Arteries

Arterial blood pressure usually declines during the second trimester due to peripheral vasodilatation caused by estrogens and prostaglandins.

The posture of the pregnant woman affects arterial blood pressure.

Typically, it is highest when she is sitting, lowest when lying in the lateral recumbent position and intermediate when supine.

Supine Hypotensive Syndrome

May develop in some women late in pregnancy in supine position.

This is due to compression of the inferior vena cava by the large pregnant uterus resulting in decrease venous return, decrease cardiac output and low blood pressure that fainting may occur.

Veins

Varicosities in the lower limbs and vulva may occur due to:

– Back pressure from the compressed inferior vena cava by the pregnant uterus.

– Relaxation of the smooth muscles in the wall of the veins by progesterone.

RESPIRATORY CHANGES

Dysponea may occur due to:

– Increase sensitivity of the respiratory center to CO_2 possibly due to high progesterone level.

– Elevation of the diaphragm by the pregnant uterus.

GASTRO-INTESTINAL CHANGES

Ptyalism (Sialorrhea)

It is excessive salivation and more common in association with oral sepsis.

Gingivitis

There is increased vascularity and tendency for bleeding as well as hypertrophy of the interdental papilla.

Nausea and Vomiting

Nausea (morning sickness) and vomiting (emesis gravidarum) occur in early months.

Appetite Changes (Longing or Craving)

The pregnant woman dislikes some foods and odours while desires others.

Reduced sensitivity of the taste buds during pregnancy creates the desire for markedly sweet, sour or salt foods.

Deviation may be so extreme to the extent of eating blackboard chalk, coal or mud (pica).

Indigestion and Flatulance

This is probably due to:

– Decreased gastric acidity caused by regurgitation of alkaline secretion from the intestine to the stomach.

– Decreased gastric motility.

Hurt Burn

Due to reflux of the acidic gastric contents to the esophagus.

Gall Stones

More tendency to stone formation due to atony and delayed emptying of the gall bladder.

Constipation

Due to:

– Reduced motility of large intestine (progesterone effect).

– Increased water reabsorption from the large intestine (aldosterone effect).

– Pressure on the pelvic colon by the pregnant uterus.

– Sedentary life during pregnancy.

Hemorroids

Due to:

- Mechanical pressure on the pelvic veins.

- Laxity of the veins walls by progesterone.

- Constipation.

Appendix

It is displaced upwards by the enlarged uterus.

URINARY CHANGES

Kidney

Renal blood flow and glomerular filtration rate increases by 50%.

Ureters

Dilatation of the ureters and renal pelvis due to:

- Relaxation of the ureters by the effect of progesterone and relaxin.

- Hypertrophy of the lower end of the ureter by the effect of estrogen.

- Pressure against the pelvic brim by the uterus particularly on the right side.

Bladder

Frequency of micturition in early pregnancy due to:

- Pressure on the bladder by the enlarged uterus.

- Congestion of the bladder mucosa.

Urinary stress incontinence may develop for the first time during pregnancy and spontaneously relieved later on.

METABOLIC CHANGES

Carbohydrate Metabolism

Pregnancy is potentially diabetogenic.

Alimentary glucosuria may occur in early pregnancy.

Renal glucosuria may occur in the middle of pregnancy.

Fasting hypoglycemia due to transfer of glucose to the fetus.

Protein Metabolism

There is tendency to nitrogen retention for fetal and maternal tissues formation.

Fat Metabolism

There is increase in plasma lipids with tendency to acidosis.

Mineral Metabolism

There is increased demand for iron, calcium, phosphate and magnesium.

Water Metabolism

There is tendency to water retention secondary to sodium retention.

Weight Gain

The average weight gain in pregnancy is 10-12 kg.

This increase occurs mainly in the second and third trimesters at a rate of 350-400 gm/week.

Six kg of the average 11 kg weight gain is composed of maternal tissues (breast, fat, blood and uterine tissue) and 5 kg of fetus, placenta and amniotic fluid.

Of this 11 kg, 7 kg are water, 3 kg fat and 1 kg protein.

ENDOCRINE SYSTEM

Pituitary Gland

The anterior pituitary enlarges due to an increase in prolactin secreting cells (lactotrophs).

Thyroid Gland

There is diffuse slight enlargement of the gland.

Gland activity increases as evidenced by the increase in:

– Basal metabolic rate (BMR) by about 30%.

– Thyroxine-binding globulin, total T3 and T4.

– Protein bound iodine (PBI).

Parathyroid Glands

Increase in size and activity to regulate increased calcium metabolism.

Adrenal Glands

Hypertrophy particularly the cortex resulting in increased mineralocorticoids (aldosterone) and glucocorticoids (cortisol).

SKELETAL CHANGES

Progressive lordosis to compensate for the anterior position of the enlarged uterus.

Increased mobility of the pelvic joints due to softening of the joints and ligaments caused by progesterone and relaxin.

OBSTETRIC HISTORY AND EXAMINATION

OBSTETRIC HISTORY

Present Obstetric History

– Calculate Expected Delivery Date (EDD = LMP + 9 months + 7 days).

– Calculate duration of pregnancy.

– Symptoms of pregnancy.

– Warning symptoms.

– Investigations done during pregnancy.

– Medications taken during pregnancy.

Past Obstetric History

– Previous miscarriages.

– Previous viable pregnancies.

– Method of delivery.

– Gestational age and sex.

– Previous antenatal or postnatal complications.

Medical History

– Hypertension.

– Diabetes.

– Cardiac disease.

– Renal disease.

– Infectious disease (e.g. Hepatitis B or C, HIV ...).

OBSTETRIC EXAMINATION

General Examination

– Vital signs.

– Weight and height.

– Stature and gait.

– CVS: flow murmurs.

– Breasts and nipples.

Abdominal Examination

– Fundal level.

– Leopold maneuvers.

– Auscultation of fetal heart sounds.

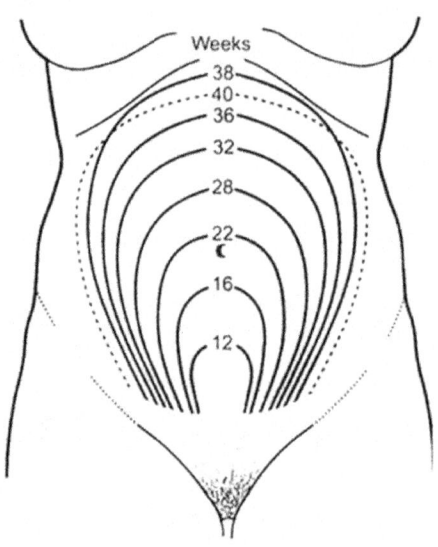

Fundal Level

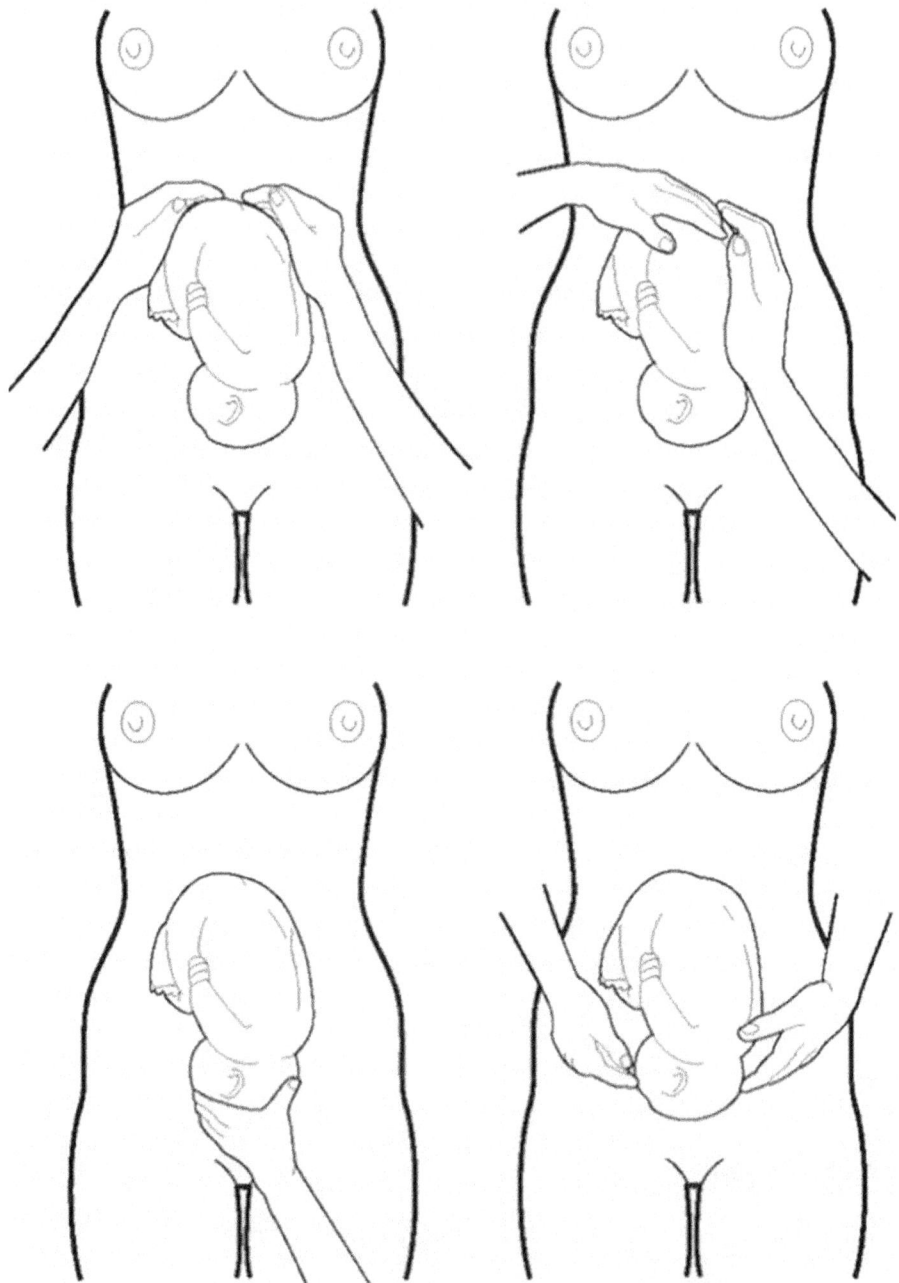

Leopold Maneuvers

DIAGNOSIS OF PREGNANCY

FIRST TRIMESTER (0-12 WEEKS)

Symptoms

Amenorrhea

Sudden cessation of a previously regular menstruation is the most common symptom denoting pregnancy.

However, pregnancy may occur during lactational amenorrhea.

On the other hand, bleeding may occur early in pregnancy as in threatened abortion.

Slight bleeding may occur also at the expected time of menstruation in the first 12 weeks of pregnancy but never afterwards due to separation of parts of the decidua vera.

Morning Sickness

Nausea with or without vomiting commences in the morning.

It usually appears about 6 weeks after onset of the last menstrual period and usually disappears 6-12 weeks later.

Frequency of Micturition

Due to congestion and pressure on the bladder and disappear after the first trimester to reappear again near the end of pregnancy when the fetal head descends into the maternal pelvis.

Breast Symptoms

Enlargement, sensation of fullness, tingling and tenderness.

Appetite Changes

Longing or Craving

Signs

Breast Signs

– Increase in size and vascularity.

– Increase pigmentation of the nipple and primary areola.

– Appearance of the secondary areola.

– Montgomery's follicles.

– Expression of colostrum.

Breast signs are diagnostic only in primigravidae.

Uterine Signs

The uterus becomes enlarged, globular and soft.

Hegar's sign (6-10weeks): During bimanual examination, the two fingers in the anterior fornix can be approximated to fingers of the abdominal hand behind the uterus due to softening and emptiness of the lower part of the uterus.

Palmer's Sign: Uterine contractions felt during bimanual examination.

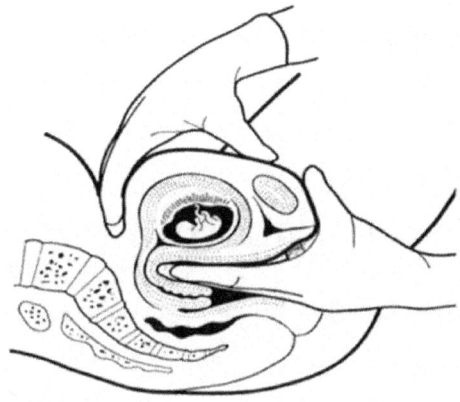

Hegar's Sign

Cervix

Soft, hypertrophied and violet.

Vagina

Violet, moist, warm with increased acidity.

Investigations

Pregnancy Tests

These depend on presence of human chorionic gonadotrophin (hCG) in maternal serum and urine.

Urine Pregnancy Tests

Rapid and simple tests.

Based on enzyme-labelled monoclonal antibodies assay.

Can detect low level of hCG in urine.

Causes of false positive results:

− Proteinuria.

− Hematuria.

− At time of ovulation (cross reaction with LH).

− hCG injection for infertility treatment within the previous 30 days.

− Thyrotoxicosis (high TSH).

− Premature menopause (high LH and FSH).

− Early days after delivery or abortion.

− Trophoblastic diseases.

− hCG secreting tumors.

Causes of false negative results:

– Too early pregnancy.

– Missed abortion.

– Ectopic pregnancy.

– Urine stored too long in room temperature.

– Interfering medications.

Serum Pregnancy Tests

It is the earliest available method for accurate diagnosis of pregnancy.

– Radioimmunoassay of B-hCG.

– Radio receptor assay.

– Enzyme-linked immunosorbent assay (ELISA).

Sensitivity of pregnancy tests:

	Lowest hCG (mIU/ml)	Minimum day (postovulatory)
Urine		
- Slide	500-2500	17-26
- Tube	75-1000	14-22
Serum		
- Radioimmunoassay	300-500	9
- Radiorecepter	100-200	9
- ELISA	50	7-10

Serum B-hCG is superior to urine pregnancy test in the early diagnosis of normal pregnancy, and in the follow up of abnormal pregnancy since it is a quantitative test with high sensitivity and extremely low false positive results.

Uses of pregnancy test:

– Diagnosis of pregnancy.

– Diagnosis of fetal death.

– Diagnosis of ectopic pregnancy.

– Diagnosis and follow up of gestational trophoblastic diseases.

The pregnancy test becomes negative about:

– 1 week after labor.

– 2 weeks after abortion.

– 4 weeks after evacuation of vesicular mole.

Ultrasonography

– Gestational sac can be detected after 5 weeks of amenorrhea.

– Fetal heart pulsation can be detected as early as 7 weeks.

– Fetal crown to rump length (CRL) in the first trimester.

– Biparietal diameter (BPD), abdominl circumference (AC) and femur length (FL) in the second trimester.

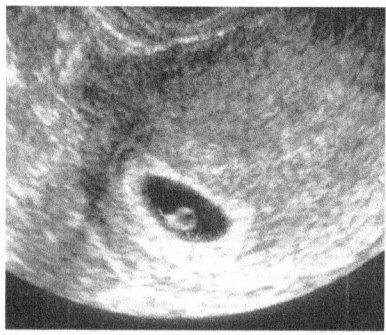 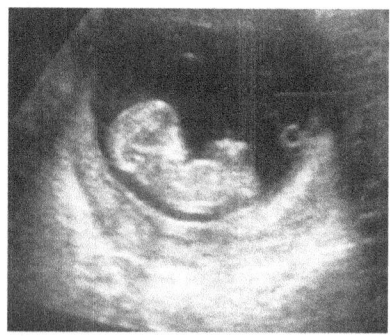

Early Pregnancy Ultrasonography

SECOND TRIMESTER (13-28 WEEKS)

Symptoms

– Amenorrhea.

– Morning sickness and urinary symptoms decrease.

– Quickening: The first sensation of the fetal movement by the mother, occurs at 18-20 weeks in primigravida and at 16-18 weeks in multiparas.

– Abdominal enlargement.

Signs

Breast Signs

Become more manifested.

Uterine Signs

The uterus is felt abdominally.

Braxton Hick's contractions: intermittent painless contractions can be felt by abdominal examination.

Palpation of fetal parts and movement: by the obstetrician at 20 weeks.

Fetal heart sound: can be auscultated at 20-24 weeks by the Pinard's stethoscope.

Umbilical (funic) souffle: A murmur with the same rate of FHS due to rush of blood in the umbilical arteries, occasionally detected when a loop of the cord lies below the stethoscope.

Internal ballottement: at 16 weeks by a push to the fetal parts with the two fingers through the anterior fornix.

External ballottement: at 20 weeks by a push to the fetal parts with one hand abdominally and the other hand receiving the impulse.

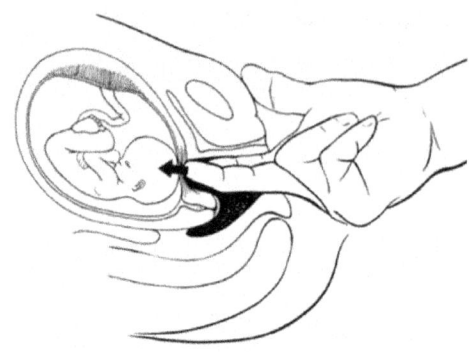

Internal Ballottement

Investigations

Pregnancy tests are positive.

Ultrasonography is diagnostic.

THIRD TRIMESTER (29-40 WEEKS)

All signs of pregnancy become more evident.

Pregnancy tests are positive.

Ultrasonography is diagnostic.

Sure Signs of Pregnancy

– Inspection of fetal movements.

– Palpation of fetal parts.

– Palpation of fetal movements.

– Auscultation of fetal heart sounds.

– The occasional auscultation of the umbilical (funic) souffle.

– Ultrasonographic detection of fetal parts, movements and/or heart movements.

Differential Diagnosis of Pregnancy

<u>Early Pregnancy</u>

Causes of amenorrhea.

Causes of symmetrically enlarged uterus:

– Myoma.

– Adenomyosis.

– Pyometra.

– Hematometra.

– Metropathia hemorrhagica.

Pelvi-abdominal swellings:

– Ovarian swellings.

– Tubal swellings.

– Pelvic hematocele.

– Full bladder.

<u>Late Pregnancy</u>

– Myomas.

– Ovarian neoplasm.

– Ascitis.

– Pseudocyesis.

– Other causes of pelvi-abdominal mass.

ANTENATAL CARE

OBJECTIVES

– Prevention, early detection and treatment of pregnancy related complications as pre-eclampsia, eclampsia and hemorrhage.

– Prevention, early detection and treatment of medical disorders as anemia and diabetes.

– Detection of malpresentations, malpositions and disproportion that may influence the decision of labor.

– Instruct the pregnant woman about hygiene, diet and warning symptoms.

– Laboratory studies of parameters may affect the fetus as blood group, Rh typing, toxoplasmosis and syphilis.

PRECONCEPTION VISIT

The ideal first visit should be at a preconception clinic where health education and risk assessment can be directed towards the planned pregnancy.

Advice can be given regarding the avoidance of harmful and teratogenic factors (drugs, cigarette smoking and alcohol intake…), ensuring an optimal dietary intake, and absence or control of chronic medical disorders (as diabetes, hypertension…), in order to allow pregnancy to be started in the optimum conditions.

FREQUENCY OF ANTENATAL VISITS

– Every month during the first 6 months.

– Every 2 weeks during the 7th and 8th months.

– Every week during the last month.

– More frequent visits are indicated in high risk pregnancy.

FIRST VISIT

History: Menstrual, obstetric, medical, surgical, and family history.

Examination: General, abdominal and local.

Laboratory investigations

– Blood grouping.

– Rh typing.

– Hemoglobin.

– Urine analysis particularly for albumin and sugar.

– Toxoplasma and/or VDRL if needed.

RETURN VISITS

History: Ask the patient about any complaint.

Examination

– Blood pressure.

– Weight.

– Edema.

– Abdominal examination.

Investigation: Urine for albumin and sugar, and ultrasonography if needed.

INSTRUCTIONS TO PREGNANT WOMAN

Rest and Sleep: 2 hours in the mid-day and 8 hours at night.

Exercises: Violent exercises as diving and water sports should be avoided. House work short of fatigue and walking are encouraged.

Travelling

Long and tiring journeys should be avoided particularly if the woman is prone to abortion or preterm labor.

Flying is not contraindicated but not the long ones and near term.

Bathing: Shower bathing is preferable than tube or sea bathing for fear of ascending infection. Vaginal douching should be avoided.

Bowels: Constipation is avoided by increasing vegetables, fluids and milk intake and mild exercise. Liquid paraffin should not be used for long period as it interferes with absorption of fat-soluble vitamins (A and D).

Teeth: Regular cleansing. Consult the dentist when needed.

Clothing:

Lighter and looser clothes of non synthetic materials are more comfortable due to increased BMR and sweating.

Clothes which hang from the shoulders are more comfortable than that requiring waste bands.

Breast support is required.

Shoes: High-heeled shoes should be discouraged as they increase lumbar lordosis, back strain and risk of falling.

Breasts: to reduce the incidence of retracted and/or cracked nipples postpartum, the patient is instructed to massage them with a mixture of glycerine and alcohol during the last 6 weeks of pregnancy.

Coitus

Whenever abortion or preterm labor is a threat, coitus should be avoided.

Otherwise, it is allowed with less frequency and violence.

Some obstetricians advise abstinence in the last 4 weeks of pregnancy for fear of ascending infection.

Diet

The daily requirements are:

– Calories: 2500 Kcal.

– Proteins: 60 gm.

– Carbohydrates: 200-400 gm.

– Lipids: should be restricted.

Vitamins

– Vitamin A: 5000 IU.

– Vitamin B1 (Thiamine): 1mg.

– Vitamin B2 (Riboflavin): 1.5 mg.

– Nicotinic acid: 15mg.

– Ascorbic acid (vit. C): 50mg.

– Vitamin D: 400 IU.

– Folic acid: 0.5 mg.

Minerals

– Iron: 15 mg.

– Calcium: 1000 mg.

So the suggested daily diet should include:

– 1 litre of milk or its derivatives,

– 1-2 eggs.

– 2 pieces of red meat replaced once weekly by sea fish and once by calf's liver.

– Fresh vegetables and fruits.

– Cereals and bread are recommended also.

– Coffee and tea: should be restricted.

Effect of Malnutrition on Pregnancy

Effect on the Mother

– Loss of weight and anaemia.

– Decalcification of bones, caries of teeth.

– Postpartum haemorrhage.

– Affection of lactation.

– Lowered resistance against infection.

Effect on the Fetus

– Abortion and preterm labor.

– Intrauterine fetal death.

– Low birth weight infants.

– Higher incidence of rickets and anaemia, in severe cases.

Smoking: should be avoided as it may cause intrauterine growth retardation or premature labor.

Exposure to Infections: is to be avoided particularly those of documented teratogenicity e.g. rubella, cytomegalovirus, herpes hominis and varicella zoster viruses.

Exposure to Irradiation: is to be avoided whether diagnostic or therapeutic.

Medications: not to be taken without obstetrician advice due to risk of teratogenicity.

Drug Categories during Pregnnacy (FDA Classification)

– Group A: Safe during pregnancy.

– Group B: Risky in animal, no enough data on humans.

– Group C: Risk in human cannot be ruled out.

– Group D: Risky in human pregnancy, but benefits may outweigh risks.

– Group X: Contraindicated, may cause adverse fetal effects.

Immunisation

Nature of Vaccine	Name	Allowance
Live virus vaccines	Measles	Contraindicated.
	Mumps	Contraindicated.
	Rubella	Contraindicated.
	Poliomyelitis	In risk of exposure only.
	Yellow fever	Travel to endemic areas.
Inactivated virus vaccines	Influenza	Serious underlying disease.
	Rabies	Same as non-pregnant.
Inactivated bacterial vaccines	Cholera	For international travels.
	Typhoid fever	Travel to endemic areas.
	Plague	Selective for exposed persons.
	Meningococcal meningitis	Same as non-pregnant.
Toxoid	Tetanus	Same as non-pregnant.
	Diphtheria	
Immune globulins	Rabies	Post-exposure prophylaxis.
	Tetanus	
	Varicella	
	Measles	
	Hepatitis A	
	Hepatitis B	Post-exposure prophylaxis along with hepatitis B vaccine initially, then vaccine alone at 1 and 6 months.

Warning Symptoms: which indicate immediate contact to the obstetrician are:

– Persistent headache.

– Blurring of vision.

– Persistent vomiting.

– Abdominal pain.

– Dimineshed fetal movements.

– Vaginal bleaeding.

– Gush of fluid per vagina.

– Edema of lower limbs or face.

MINOR COMPLAINTS DURING PREGNANCY

GASTRO-INTESTINAL

Ptyalism (Sialorrhea)

Increased salivation may occur early in pregnancy and subsides later on.

It is due to failure of the patient to swallow the saliva rather than increase in its amount.

Treatment

– Care of dental hygiene.

– Discontinue smoking.

– Anticholinergic drugs as belladonna, which induce dryness of the mouth, may be needed.

Gingivitis

Increased vascularity and hypertrophy of the interdental papillae.

Sequelae

– Increased tendency for bleeding.

– Retention of food debris predisposes to sepsis and dental caries.

Treatment

– Proper dental hygiene.

– Cryosurgery for severe cases.

Nausea and Vomiting

Nausea (morning sickness) and vomiting (emesis gravidarum) occur in early months.

Heartburn

A common complaint caused by reflux of gastric contents into the lower esophagus due to mechanical relaxation of the cardiac sphincter caused by upward displacement and compression of the stomach by the pregnant uterus.

Treatment

– More frequent but smaller meals.

– Avoidance of bending over or lying flat.

– Antacids containing aluminium hydroxide are preferable as they buffer the gastric contents, do not cause an acid rebound and not absorbed so that alkalosis is unlikely.

Constipation

Causes

– Reduced intestinal motility due to steroid hormones.

– Increased fluid resorption from the large bowel.

– Reduced exercise.

– Mechanical compression by the gravid uterus.

Treatment

– Evacuate the bowel at the same time every day.

– Increase fluid intake.

– Diet rich in green vegetables, bran and fruits.

– Mild laxative as senna preparations.

– Liquid paraffin interferes with absorption of fat soluble vitamins, so better to be avoided.

Hemorrhoids

Causes

– Laxity of the rectal veins by progesterone effect.

– Pressure by the gravid uterus.

– Tendency to constipation.

Treatment

– Avoid constipation.

– Soothing and astringent agents.

– Local anesthetics.

– Surgical and local injection treatment should be avoided.

RESPIRATORY

Dyspnea

It may occur early in pregnancy due to hyperventilation caused by progesterone.

Late in pregnancy, it occurs due to pressure on the diaphragm by the pregnant uterus.

URINARY

Frequency and stress incontinence may occur during pregnancy.

Causes

– Increased intra-abdominal pressure.

– Pressure on the bladder by the enlarging uterus reducing its capacity.

Urinary tract infection should be excluded.

GENITAL

Leucorrhea

Increased vaginal discharge is a common complaint during pregnancy due to excess estrogen production.

No treatment is needed except if there is associated infection.

Monilial infection is common.

VASCULAR

Varicosities

Varicose veins may occur in the vulva and/or lower limbs.

In addition to the non-cosmetic appearance, they cause edema, discomfort and even ulcers, dermatitis and superficial thrombophlebitis.

Causes

Congenital weakness which are exaggerated by:

– Increased venous pressure by compression with the pregnant uterus.

– Prolonged standing.

– Relaxation of veins walls by steroid hormones.

Treatment

– Avoid prolonged standing.

– Encourage active exercise.

– Elevate the legs during sitting and sleeping.

– Elastic stocking are worn while the patient is lying down and veins are empty.

– Surgical or injection treatment should be avoided during pregnancy.

NEUROLOGICAL

Paraethesia

Tingling sensation of the fingers and sometimes weakness of small muscles of the hand.

Causes

– Edema of the carpal tunnel which may be relieved by diuretics.

– Brachial plexus traction due to shoulder dropping during pregnancy.

MUSCULO-SKELETAL

Leg Cramps

Causes

– Depletion of serum calcium as well as sodium and chloride.

– Local vascular insufficiency.

Management

– Massage of the contracted muscles and passive stretching.

– Calcium gluconate may be helpful.

Backache

Causes

– Lumbar lordosis.

– Relaxation of ligaments and intervertebral joints by progesterone effect.

Management

– Adequate rest and support the back when sitting in a chair by a pillow.

– Avoid wearing high-heeled shoes.

HIGH RISK PREGNANCY

DEFINITTION

High risk pregnancy is a pregnancy complicated by a disease or a disorder that may affect the health or endanger the life of the mother or the fetus.

IDENTIFICATION

High risk pregnancy is identified by proper assessment through history, clinical examination and special investigations.

History

– Age: whether young (<18) or elderly (>35) primigravida.

– Parity: whether nullipara or grand multipara.

– Previous obstetric difficulties, fetal loss or abnormalities.

– Medical disorders as: diabetes, cardiac or renal disease.

General Examination

– Extreme obesity and short stature.

– Hypertension.

– Severe anemia, cardiac or renal disease.

– Poor weight gain during pregnancy.

Obstetric Examination

– Preeclampsia.

– Antepartum hemorrhage.

– Multiple pregnancy.

– Malpresentations and fetopelvic disproportion.

Investigations

– Severe anemia, thrombocytopaenia and hyperglycaemia.

– Glycosuria and albuminuria.

– Rh negative blood typing.

Screening for Fetal Anomalies

– Congenital anomalies: e.g. anencephay, NTDs, limb and skeletal deformities, cardiac and renal anomalies, etc… by ultrasonography for fetal anatomy survey.

– Chromosomal anomalies: as Down's syndrome (by 1st trimester ultrasonography, chorionic villus sampling, and 2nd trimester amniocentesis).

Screening for Infections

– TORCH, toxoplasmosis, rubella, cytomegalovirus, herpes simplex.

– Hepatitis B and C and HIV.

MANAGEMENT

Preconception Counseling

The obstetrician discusses and explains the following items:

– The high risk factor(s) and its possible effects on the mother, fetus, and the newborn.

– The importance of proper monitoring during pregnancy and labor.

– The possibility of early intervention and the sequelae of preterm labor.

– The need for antenatal care in a well equipped antenatal clinic.

– The need to deliver in a well equipped hospital, with warning against home delivery.

Antenatal Care

Once identified during preconception visit, first antenatal visit or return visits, the mother should be transferred for antenatal care and delivery in a specialized center ready for such high risk cases.

Fetal Surveillance

- Correlation between fetal growth and gestational age (clinical and ultrasonography).

- Daily Fetal Movement Count (DFMC).

- Non stress test (NST).

- Contraction stress test (CST).

- Biophysical profile (BPP) score.

- Doppler ultrasonography.

Delivery of High Risk Patients

- Attention to the risks that may develop during labor and may affect maternal or fetal conditions.

- The place of delivery should be fully equipped for maternal and fetal resuscitation (maternal and neonatal ICU).

- Efficient well-trained personnel, specialists and consultants should be available 24 hours a day.

- Monitoring of fetal well being during labor, maternal condition and progress of labor (partogram) is essential.

Postnatal Care

- The mother is still at risk for complications during the immediate and late postpartum period.

- The new born must be assessed and managed by a neonatologist.

ELDERLY PRIMIGRAVIDA

Definition

Primigravida whose age is 35 years or more during pregnancy or delivery.

Maternal and Fetal Risks

– Medical disorders: Pregnancy induced hypertension and diabetes.

– Intrauterine growth retardation and preterm labor.

– Chromosomal anomalies (triosmy 21) and congenital malformations.

– Uterine inertia and rigid perineum.

– Increased incidence of operative delivery and cesarean section.

GRAND MULTIPARA

Definition

Women who had 5 or more previous deliveries.

Maternal and Fetal Risks

– Medical disorders: Pregnancy induced hypertension, diabetes and anemia.

– Placenta previa and placenta accretaq.

– Malpresentations due to pendulous abdomen.

– Uterine inertia, prolonged labor, premature rupture of membranes and prolapsed cord.

– Obstructed labor and rupture uterus.

– Increased incidence of operative delivery and cesarean section.

– Postpartum hemorrhage, puerperal sepsis and subinvolution.

MATERNAL MORTALITY

Definitions

Maternal Mortality

Maternal deaths due to obstetric causes (during pregnancy, delivery, or puerperium).

Maternal Mortality Rate (MMR)

Number of maternal deaths due to obstetric causes per 100,000 deliveries per year.

Causes

- Postpartum hemorrhage.

- Pregnancy induced hypertension.

- Antepartum haemorrhage.

- Infection: Post-partum and post-abortive.

- Rupture of the uterus.

- Complications of cesarean section.

- Pulmonary embolism and DIC.

- Medical problems as heart disease with pregnancy.

- Complications of anaesthesia.

FETAL/NEONATAL MORTALITY

Definitions

Intrauterine Fetal Death

Fetal death during pregnancy.

Intrapartum Fetal Death

Fetal death during delivery.

Neonatal Death

Infant death in the first 4 weeks after delivery.

Perinatal Mortality

Intrauterine fetal death + intrapartum fetal death + neonatal death during the first week after delivery.

Causes

Intrauterine Fetal Death

– Hypertensive disorders of pregnancy.

– Diabetes with pregnancy.

– Placental insufficiency.

– Rh incompatibility.

– Congenital fetal anomalies.

– True knots of the cord.

– Idiopathic (unexplained).

Intrapartum Fetal Death

– Asphyxia.

– Birth trauma.

– Intracranial hemorrhage.

– Intra-amniotic infection.

Neonatal Death

– Prematurity.

– Neonatal asphyxia.

– Birth injuries.

– Congenital fetal anomalies.

– Hemolytic and hemorrhagic diseases of the newly born.

– Respiratory distress syndrome.

– Neonatal infection.

REFERENCES

– Abalos E, Chamillard M, Diaz V, et al. Antenatal care for healthy pregnant women: a mapping of interventions from existing guidelines to inform the development of new WHO guidance on antenatal care. BJOG. 2016; 123: 519.

– ACOG Committee Opinion. Clinical Management Guidelines for Obstetrician-Gynecologists. Number 88. 2007.

– ACOG Committee Opinion. Preconception care. Number 313. 2015.

– Attilakos G, Overton T. Antenatal Care, in Dewhurst's Textbook of Obstetrics & Gynaecology. 8th ed. Oxford, UK: Wiley-Blackwell; 2012.

– Berek J, Adashi E, Hillard P. Novak's Gynecology. 14th ed. Baltimore, MD: Lippincott Williams & Wilkins; 2006.

– Chard T. Pregnancy tests: a review. Hum Reprod 1992; 7: 701.

– Chung K. Gross Anatomy. 4th ed. Philadelphia, PA: Lippincott Williams & Wilkins; 2000.

– Cole L. Human chorionic gonadotropin tests. Expert Rev Mol Diagn 2009; 9: 721.

– Cunningham F, MacDonald P, Gant N. Williams Obstetrics. 19th ed. Norwalk, Conn: Appleton & Lange; 1993.

– Drake R, Vogl A, Mitchell A. Gray's Anatomy for Student's. 2nd ed. Philadelphia, PA: Churchill Livingstone Elsevier; 2010.

– Foxcroft K, Callaway L, Byrne N, et al. Development and validation of a pregnancy symptoms inventory. BMC Pregnancy Childbirth. 2013; 13: 3.

– Gray H. Anatomy, Descriptive and Surgical. The Unabridged Gray's Anatomy. Philadelphia, PA: Running Press; 1999.

– Guyton and hall. Textbook of Medical Physiology. 11 ed. Philadelphia, PA: Saunders; 2005.

– Junqueira L, Carneiro J, Kelley R. Basic Histology. 9th ed. Stamford, Connecticut: Appleton & Lange; 1998.

– Katz V, Lentz G, Lobo R, et al. Comprehensive Gynecology. 5th ed. Philadelphia, PA: Mosby Elsevier; 2007.

– Loukas M, Colburn G, Abrahams P, et al. Gray's Anatomy Review. Philadelphia, PA: Churchill Livingstone Elsevier; 2010.

– Moore K, Persaud T. The Developing Human: Clinically Oriented Embryology. 5th ed. Philadelphia, PA: WB Saunders; 1993.

– Neill J. Knobil and Neill's Physiology of Reproduction. 3rd ed. St. Louis, MO: Elsevier; 2006.

– Ovalle W, Nahirney P. Netter's Eseential Histology. Philadelphia, PA: Sauders Elsevier; 2007.

– Practice Bulletin No. 175: Ultrasound in Pregnancy. Obstet Gynecol. 2016; 128: e241.

– Sadler T. Langman's Medical Embryology. 11th ed. Baltimore, Maryland: Lippincott Williams & Wilkins; 2010.

– Speroff L, Fritz M. Clinical Gynecologic Endocrinology and Infertility. 7th ed. Philadelphia, PA: Lippincott Williams & Wilkins; 2005.

– Standring S. Gray's Anatomy. 40th ed. Edinburgh: Elsevier Churchill Livingstone; 2008.